Bath Bombs Book

Natural and Organic Homemade Bath Bombs Beginner's Guide

T.A. Krauss

Table of Contents

Chapter 1: Introduction

Bath bombs are balls that fizz and create bubbles when dropped into water. They vary in size and shape. They make you relax due to the scents and bubbles that turn your bathtub to a mini-spa.

They are fit for everyone and fit every occasion provided you have a bathtub. They are cheap to make and this will save you some pennies and time shopping.

This book will guide you on how to make bath bombs. You will visualize the steps so that you can jumpstart your own creativity and come up with wonderful recipes of your own.

Hopefully, you will enjoy every word of the book. Doing it practically is the blow.

BackToTop

Conversion Table

- 1/2 fl oz = 3 tsp = 1 tbsp = 15 ml
- 1 fl oz = 2 tbsp = 1/8 c = 30 ml
- 2 fl oz = 4 tbsp = 3/4 c = 60 ml
- 4 fl oz = 8 tbsp = 1/2 c = 118 ml
- 8 fl oz = 16 tbsp = 1 c = 236 ml
- 16 fl oz = 1 pt = 1/2 qt = 2 c = 473 ml
- 128 fl oz = 8 pt = 4 qt = 1 gal = 3.78 L

Abbreviations

- oz = ounce
- fl oz = fluid ounce
- tsp = teaspoon
- tbsp = tablespoon
- ml = milliliter
- c = cup
- pt = pint
- qt = quart
- gal = gallon
- L = liter

Chapter 2: Bath Bomb Basics

Bath bombs are easy to make. The number of ingredients depends on the kind of bath bomb you want to make. The main principles you need to know are the key ingredients, getting the right consistency, molding, adding extras, storage and presentation.

Key Ingredients

Fizzing is the key thing. What makes bath bombs fizz? There are really only two ingredients that make fizzing happen: citric acid and baking soda. When a mixture is dropped into water, these two ingredients react to create lots of lovely bubbles.

If you still can't find any citric acid, the easiest alternative is to use cream of tartar. Cream of tartar is stronger than citric acid, so a general rule of thumb is to use, replace citric acid in a recipe and use half the amount of cream of tartar. The ratio of baking soda to citric acid should always be 1; 2. If you're using cream of tartar instead of citric acid, then the ratio of baking soda to cream of tartar will be 1;1.

The Right Consistency

Getting the right consistency can be challenging, ingredients used can react in many different ways giving unpleasant results. The humidity of the area around you could also affect the consistency of the mixture.

The trick, though, is the texture of the mixture, that way you know when to start molding. You can check for consistency by packing the mixture between your hands. The bath bomb should feel damp sandy so that it clumps together. If it is sticky like Play-Doh and feels really wet, then you have put in too much liquid. You need to add more dry ingredients. However, if it doesn't stay clumped for very long, and crumbles easily, or it feels hard and pebbly, you will need to add more liquid because the mixture is too dry.

The key to getting the right consistency is to add ingredients in slowly. Adding too much of either dry or liquid ingredients at a time, makes it difficult to achieve the perfect texture.

Molding

The mold you use determines the shape of your bath bomb. You can get a variety of shapes using anything. One option is to buy bath bomb molds sold in craft stores. A cheaper alternative would be using anything you already have in the house. These could be baking molds, muffin tins, and plastic candy.

The mixture needs to be packed in tightly to prevent them from cracking. This can be done by putting in only little quantities at a time.

Keep doing this until you've filled the mold to the top. You'll then need to remove them to dry. To do this, gently turn the mold over and tap the bath bombs out.

Adding Extras

You can add a variety of ingredients to give a bath bomb a particular look or fragrance. Here a few ways to add extra ingredients into your bath bomb mixture:

- **Liquid Ingredients**: Food coloring, perfumes, fragrances and essential oils are common additions to bath bombs. They should be mixed in with the liquid ingredients before combining with the dry ingredients.

- **Dry ingredients**: Extras like dried petals, nut and glitter can be added to the other dry ingredients in the recipe before you add in the liquid ingredients. They could be crushed and powdered or in sizable chunks

- **Decorative Ingredients**: you may prefer to put decorative items on the bath bomb to inside it. Place the ingredient such as glitter, lavender buds or rosehips into the bottom of the mold before packing the mixture in. When you remove the bath bomb, the decorative items will be on top.

Caution: when customizing your bath bombs, remember that they will be used in a bathtub. Try to avoid anything that may cause an allergy or skin reaction. For instance, if you know someone that has a nut allergy, don't include nuts or nut oils in your bath bomb mixture.

Avoid ingredients that may react with your key ingredients. Try to stay away from acids like vinegar (vinegar doesn't really smell good anyway) and it may also affect the 2:1 ratio of your baking soda to citric acid.

Try some of the special recipes in this book to customize your bath bombs more.

Storage and Presentation

Store bath bomb sin a cool dry place. They are highly vulnerable to humidity and heat. Airtight containers are ideal for keeping bath bombs.

One of the best ways for storing bath bombs for whichever reason is in glass jars. You can decorate the jars with ribbons, paint, glitter or bits of colored paper to give them a truly personal touch. Glass jars are also non-reactive, so you won't need to worry about your bath bombs undergoing a chemical reaction during storage.

You could also seal the bath bombs in airtight sandwich bags.

BackToTop

Chapter 3: Simple Bath Bomb Recipes

In this chapter, you will learn the two basic recipes for making bath bombs, with and without using citric acid. Any other bath bombs can be made by putting your own spin on these two recipes.

Basic Bath Bomb

Ingredients:

- 2 cups of baking soda
- 1 cup citric acid
- 1 cup Epsom salts
- 1 teaspoon water
- 3 tablespoons light vegetable oil

Directions:

1. Mix the baking soda, citric acid and Epsom salts together in a bowl, making sure you have a fairly smooth consistency without lumps.
2. Mix the oil and water in a separate bowl.

3. Slowly add the liquid mixture into the dry mixture, using a whisk to blend them together. If your mixture starts to foam, that means you're adding the liquid in too quickly.
4. Squeeze the mixture into a ball to check the consistency. It should feel like damp sand, clumping together.
5. Pack the mixture tightly into molds, using your hands or the back of a spoon and allow them to set for a few minutes.
6. Gently tap the bath bombs out of the molds and leave overnight to dry.

Basic Bath Bomb without Citric Acid

Ingredients:

- 2 cups baking soda
- ½ cup cream of tartar
- Water
- Essential oil (optional)
- Food coloring (optional)

Directions:

1. Mix the baking soda and cream of tartar in a bowl. If desired, add the food coloring and essential oil and mix it in thoroughly.
2. Add water to the mixture, mixing only 1 teaspoon at a time.
3. Squeeze the mixture after each teaspoon to check the consistency. If it clumps together in your hand, then the mixture is ready. If the clumps begin to fall apart, add a little water.
4. Pack the mixture tightly into molds, using your hands or the back of a spoon and allow them to set for a few minutes.
5. Gently tap the bath bombs out of the molds and leave overnight to dry.

BackToTop

Chapter 4: Fragrant Bath Bomb Recipes

It's time to try some fun twists on bath bombs! One reason that bath bombs make such great gifts is that their scents often make bath time feel more relaxing. The next few recipes will help you make fabulous fragrant bath bombs.

Dried Flower Bath Bombs

Dried flower petals are a great way to give your bath bombs a light floral scent and summery feel. They also add some texture and color to the bath bomb.

Ingredients:

- Dried flower petals
- 2 cups baking soda
- 1 cup citric acid
- 1 cup cornstarch
- ½ teaspoon essential oil of your choosing
- 1 to 3 teaspoons olive oil
- 5 drops food coloring
- Spray bottle filled with water
- Round molds

Directions:

1. Mix the dried flowers, baking soda, citric acid and cornstarch in a medium-sized bowl.

2. Mix the essential oil and olive oil together in a small bowl. Add in the food coloring and mix thoroughly.
3. Slowly stir the liquid mixture into the dry ingredients, making sure the liquid is mixed in thoroughly.
4. Using the spray bottle, mist the mixture with water until it begins to feel like wet sand and clumps together in your hand.
5. Pack the bath bomb mixture tightly into the round molds.
6. Leave the bath bombs to set for a few minutes.
7. Gently turn the molds over and tap the bath bombs out.
8. Leave the bath bombs in a cool dry place for 1 to 2 days until thoroughly dry.

White Tea and Coconut Oil Bath Bombs

An interesting fact about white tea is that real estate agents actually use the scent to sell homes because it gives people a strong sense of comfort and wellbeing. Combined with the soothing scent of coconut oil, this bath bomb recipe is guaranteed to turn your bathroom into a cozy spa.

Ingredients:

- 1 cup baking soda
- ½ cup citric acid
- 2 tablespoons Epsom salts
- ½ cup cornstarch
- 2 tablespoons coconut oil
- 5 teaspoons of strong white tea
- Few drops of the essential oil of your choosing (optional)
- All-natural food coloring (optional)
- Mold
- Airtight container

Directions:

1. Mix baking soda, citric acid, Epsom salts and cornstarch in a bowl.
2. Using a whisk, work the coconut oil into the mixture until it becomes sandy with chunks of oil.
3. Mix in the white tea 1 tablespoon at a time and use a large wooden spoon to stir after

adding each teaspoon. You should expect some foam to form in the mixture after each spoon, so don't worry if this happens.

4. Keep stirring until you achieve a consistency of slightly damp sand when squeezed between your fingers.
5. Tightly pack the mixture into your mold and leave the bath bomb in the mold for at least 4 hours but preferably overnight.
6. Carefully remove the bath bombs from the mold and store them in an airtight container.

Green Tea Bath Bombs

There are few things as invigorating as green tea. Incorporating this scent into your bath bomb will make you feel refreshed and uplifted after your bath.

Ingredients:

- 2 tablespoons baking soda
- 1 tablespoon citric acid
- 1 tablespoon cornstarch

- 1 tablespoon Epsom salts
- ¼ teaspoon canola oil
- ¾ teaspoon strong green tea
- 1 or 2 drops of green food coloring

Directions:

1. Brew a strong cup of green tea. Leave it to cool to room temperature.
2. Mix the baking soda, citric acid, cornstarch and Epsom salts in bowl, using a whisk to achieve a fairly smooth consistency.
3. Mix ¾ teaspoon of the green tea with the canola oil and green food coloring in a separate bowl.
4. Slowly pour the liquid mixture into the bowl of dry ingredients, whisking to mix it in thoroughly.
5. When the mixture starts feeling like damp sand, spoon the bath bomb mixture into the molds and press in tightly.
6. Leave the bath bombs in the molds for about 4 hours.
7. Tap the bath bombs out of the mold and leave to dry for 1 to 2 days.

Coconut and Vanilla Bath Bombs

Vanilla scent is a great stress reliever and is at the same time a very alluring scent. The combination with coconut results in a bath bomb with a potent, exotic fragrance.

Ingredients:

- 2 tablespoons baking soda
- 1 tablespoon citric acid
- 1 tablespoon cornstarch
- 1 tablespoon Epsom salts
- ¼ teaspoon canola oil
- ¼ teaspoon coconut extract
- ¼ teaspoon vanilla extract
- 1 or 2 drops of blue skin-safe colorant

Directions:

1. Whisk together the baking soda, citric acid, cornstarch and Epsom salts in a bowl.
2. Mix the vanilla extract, coconut extract, canola oil and blue colorant in a different bowl.

3. Slowly drizzle the wet ingredients into the dry mixture, working the liquid in with your hands.
4. When the mixture starts to feel like damp sand and clumps together, pack it tightly into molds.
5. Leave the bath bombs in the molds for a minute or two. Then carefully pop them out onto a plush, fluffy towel on a flat surface.
6. Let the bath bombs dry for 24 to 48 hours.

Rustic Bath Bombs

Rustic bath bombs use the best natural scents of dried herbs and flowers to give you a sense of being close to nature. They lend the bath bomb a comforting feel. This recipe makes 12 bath bombs, so you can either combine all the scents into each bath bomb or make bath bombs of different scents. In this case, we'll make four different kinds of rustic bath bombs.

Ingredients:

- 10 ounces baking soda
- 6 ounces granulated citric acid
- 6 ounces cornstarch
- 6 ounces Epsom salts finely ground
- 4 teaspoons water, divided
- 4 to 8 teaspoons essential oil, divided
- 4 teaspoons extra virgin coconut oil, divided
- Food-coloring (optional)
- Dried herbs and dried flowers
- Plastic Easter egg molds
- Empty egg carton

Directions:

1. Combine the baking soda, citric acid, cornstarch and Epsom salts in a large bowl and whisk together.
2. Split the dry mixture into 4 separate bowls for each kind of scent you will be making.
3. For each bowl of dry ingredients, create a liquid mixture of 1 teaspoon of water, 1 to 2 drops of food coloring, 1to 2 teaspoons of essential oil and 1 teaspoon of coconut oil.

Make sure the wet ingredients are mixed together thoroughly.

4. Slowly add the liquid mixture into each bowl of dry ingredients and mix with a whisk.
5. When the mixture starts to bubble a little and clump together, use your fingers to work the mixture.
6. Place dried herbs and flowers in the top half of the Easter egg molds.
7. Fill both halves of the Easter egg molds with your bath bomb mixture, packing it in tightly.
8. Add a little bit of extra mixture to the top half of each Easter egg mold and press the two halves together.
9. Set the plastic eggs upright in an egg carton and leave to set for 10 minutes.
10. Turn each plastic egg upside down and gently squeeze the bottom half to remove it.
11. Place the eggs upside down in the egg carton with the top plastic half still attached and let the bath bombs dry for 2 to 4 hours.

12. Carefully place the bottom half of the plastic egg molds back on the bath bombs, and remove the top half of each egg mold.
13. Gently place the eggs right side up in the egg carton with the bottom plastic half still on and leave to dry for 4 hours.
14. Remove the bath bombs from the egg molds and place them on a plush, soft towel spread out on a flat surface. Leave to dry overnight.

Cinnamon Tea Bath Bombs

Cinnamon tea has a rich, spicy-sweet scent that brings the feel of autumn. These bath bombs infuse the air with a lovely sense of warmth.

Ingredients:

- 2 tablespoons baking soda
- 1 tablespoon citric acid
- 1 tablespoon cornstarch
- 1 tablespoon Epsom salts
- ¼ teaspoon canola oil
- ¾ teaspoon strong cinnamon tea
- 1 or 2 drops of red food coloring

Directions:

1. Brew a strong cup of cinnamon tea. Leave it to cool to room temperature.
2. While the tea is cooling, mix the baking soda, citric acid, cornstarch and Epsom salts in bowl, using a whisk to achieve a fairly smooth consistency.
3. Mix ¾ teaspoon of the green tea with the canola oil and the red food coloring in a separate bowl.
4. Slowly pour the liquid mixture into the bowl of dry ingredients, whisking to mix it in thoroughly.
5. When the mixture starts feeling like damp sand, spoon the bath bomb mixture into the molds and press in tightly.
6. Leave the bath bombs in the molds for about 4 hours.
7. Tap the bath bombs out of the mold and leave to dry for 1 to 2 days.

BackToTop

Chapter 5: Skincare Bath Bomb Recipes

Bath bombs are a wonderful way to pamper yourself and your loved ones. When you add some ingredients with skincare qualities, then you can get the added benefit of caring for your body as well. The next few recipes help you do just that.

Water Softening Bath Bombs

Hard water isn't great for long luxurious baths. Soaking in hard bathwater will often leave you with dry, itchy skin. These water softening bath bombs allow you to enjoy your long soaks in the tub.

Ingredients:

- 1 cup baking soda
- ½ cup citric acid
- ½ cup cornstarch
- 2 ½ tablespoons oil
- ¾ tablespoon water
- 2 teaspoons essential oil

- ½ teaspoon borax
- Cookie sheet

Directions:

1. Mix the baking soda, citric acid and cornstarch together in a clean bowl.
2. Mix oil, water, essential oil and borax together in a separate bowl.
3. Slowly add the liquid mixture to the dry ingredients, using one hand to squish the ingredients together.
4. When the mixture feels like damp sand, tightly pack it into the molds.
5. Let the bath bombs sit in the molds for a minute or two.
6. Flip the molds over and carefully tap the bath bombs onto a cooking sheet. Leave them to dry overnight.

Shea Butter and Citrus Bath Bombs

Shea butter is widely used in moisturizers because it's a gentle and effective skincare product. The citrus serves as a fresh scent and lends the bath bomb some astringent qualities.

Ingredients:

- 1 cup baking soda
- ½ cup citric acid
- 1 tablespoon Shea butter, melted
- 3 milliliters grapefruit essential oil
- ½ milliliter of waterless colorant
- Spray bottle with water
- Stainless steel molds

Directions:

1. Using a wire whisk, mix together the baking soda and citric acid in a bowl, breaking up any lumps in the mixture.
2. Mix the Shea butter, grapefruit essential oil and waterless colorant in a separate bowl.
3. Slowly drizzle the liquid mixture into the dry ingredients, blending the mixture together with your hands.
4. Use the spray bottle to spritz the mixture about 3 times with water. Mix together with your hands after each spritz until the mixture achieves a damp sandy consistency.

5. Scoop the mixture into the stainless steel molds, packing it in tightly with your fingers.
6. Let the bath bombs sit in the mold for a few minutes.
7. Gently tap out the bath bombs onto a cooking sheet lined with wax paper and leave to dry for 1 to 2 days in a cool, dry location away from direct heat and sunlight.

Fizzy Milk Bath Bombs

Milk baths soothe, cleanse and moisturize the skin. These fizzy milk bath bombs add a dash of fun to a luxurious skin care routine.

Ingredients:

- 1 cup baking soda
- ½ cup citric acid
- ½ cup cornstarch
- ⅓ cup Epsom salts, finely ground
- ¼ cup powdered milk
- 2 tablespoons olive oil
- 2 tablespoons cocoa butter, melted

- 1 teaspoon essential oil or fragrance oil
- Distilled water
- Witch hazel
- Spray bottle
- Molds

Directions:

1. Mix a 50/50 ratio of distilled water and witch hazel in the spray bottle and set aside.
2. Mix the baking soda, citric acid, Epsom salts and powdered milk together in a large bowl. Make sure there are no lumps.
3. Combine the olive oil, cocoa butter and essential or fragrance oil in a separate bowl.
4. Slowly drizzle the liquid mixture over the dry ingredients, using your hands to work the liquid into the mixture.
5. Using the spray bottle, mist the mixture lightly with the distilled water and witch hazel solution and mix well with your hands. Repeat until the bath bomb mixture gets the consistency of damp sand and easily clumps together.

6. Tightly pack the bath bomb mixture into your molds and leave to sit for 5 to 10 minutes.
7. Carefully remove the bath bombs from the molds and place them on a cookie sheet lined with wax paper. Let them dry for 24 to 48 hours and then store them in an airtight glass jar.

Moisture Rich Bath Bombs

One way to care for your skin is to have that extra bit of moisture that will stay on after you bathe. This recipe gives your bath bombs that added moisturizing quality.

Ingredients:

- 1 cup baking soda
- ½ cup citric acid
- ½ cup cornstarch
- ½ cup Epsom salts
- 2¾ tablespoons almond oil
- ¾ tablespoon water
- ¼ teaspoon borax
- 1½ teaspoons essential oil or fragrance oil

- Colorant
- Molds

Directions:

1. Mix the baking soda, citric acid, Epsom salts and cornstarch together.
2. Mix the almond oil, water, essential or fragrance oil, colorant and borax together in a separate bowl.
3. Slowly add the liquid mixture to the dry ingredients, whisking together as you pour.
4. When the mixture feels like damp sand, tightly pack it into the molds and leave to sit for 5 to 10 minutes.
5. Remove the bath bombs from the molds and set them on a fluffy towel. Let them dry overnight.

BackToTop

Chapter 6: Holiday-Themed Bath Bomb Recipes

Bath bombs are great gifts because they are easy to personalize and inexpensive to make. What better way to do some thoughtful gifting than with some holiday-themed bath bombs?

Christmassy Bath Bombs

Peppermint-flavored candy canes are commonly associated with Christmastime. These bath bombs have the peppermint scent and red coloring that immediately get you into the spirit of Christmas.

Ingredients:

- 8 ounces baking soda
- 4 ounces citric acid
- 4 ounces cornstarch
- 4 ounces Epsom salts
- ¾ teaspoon water
- 2 teaspoons peppermint essential oil
- 2½ teaspoons light oil (such as almond oil)
- Red food coloring
- Fillable clear plastic Christmas tree ornament ball
- Cookie sheet

- Wax paper

Directions:

1. Mix the baking soda, citric acid, cornstarch and Epson salts together in a bowl.
2. Combine the water, peppermint essential oil, light oil, and red food coloring in a small bowl.
3. Pour the liquid mixture into the dry mixture and stir with a whisk.
4. When the mixture achieves the consistency of damp sand, tightly pack the bath bomb mixture into each half of the ornament.
5. Add a little more of the mixtures on top of the second half of the ornament. Press the two halves together. If the mixture isn't packing well, simply place it back into the bowl and slowly add a little bit of water at a time. Remember, too much water will ruin the bath bomb.
6. After a few minutes, carefully remove the bath bomb from the mold.
7. Set each bath bomb on a clean cookie sheet lined with wax paper and allow to dry for at least 24 hours.

Easter Egg Bath Bombs

The pastel colored egg-shaped bath bombs are reminiscent of Easter eggs and fit right into the theme of the Easter holiday.

Ingredients:

- 8 ounces citric acid
- 8 ounces cornstarch
- 16 ounces baking soda
- 6 tablespoons almond oil
- 4 teaspoons lavender essential oil
- 3 tablespoons water
- Food coloring
- Glitter
- Plastic Easter egg molds
- Fluffy towel
- Baking sheet
- Wax paper

Directions:

1. Combine the citric acid, baking soda, cornstarch and glitter together in a large mixing bowl.

2. Whisk the almond oil, lavender essential oil and water together in a smaller bowl.
3. Add food coloring to the liquid mixture one drop at a time until you reach the desired coloring.
4. Slowly add the wet ingredients into the dry mixture, mixing together with your hands.
5. When the mixture has achieved the consistency of damp sand, fill the Easter egg molds with the bath bomb mixture, packing it in tightly.
6. Allow the bath bombs to set in the molds for several minutes.
7. Carefully remove the Easter egg bath bombs from the molds and place them on a sheet of wax paper on top of a fluffy towel. The towel ensures that the eggs do not become flat on the bottom.
8. Leave your bath bombs to dry for about 2 days.

BackToTop

Chapter 7: Specialty Bath Bomb Recipes

This chapter presents a collection of recipes that will help you create quirky, unique bath bombs. They are perfect for adding some extra fun to your bath time.

Bath Bomb Favors

Use this recipe before your party and give your guests these little bath bomb favors as they leave. Alternatively, you and your guests could easily make them together during the party and have them delivered when they are dry. This will definitely create some fun memories that will last long after the event is over. This particular recipe is tailored to wedding showers but can be slightly modified for any kind of party.

Ingredients:

- 1 cup baking soda
- ½ cup citric acid
- Spray bottle filled with witch hazel
- Essential oil or fragrance oil of your choosing
- Water free colorant
- Mini muffin pan

- Wax paper

Directions:

1. Mix the baking soda and citric acid together in a bowl with a whisk, making sure to break up any lumps.
2. Add the desired essential oil or fragrance oil to the dry mixture one or two drops at a time. The amount needed varies depending on the type of oil you are using and how strong of a scent you want. Continue adding one to two drops at a time, stirring and smelling the mixture after every drop until you reach the desired scent.
3. Add the water-free colorant one drop at a time to the mixture, stirring after each drop. If any clumps form, use your fingers to break them up.
4. Spritz the mixture with witch hazel until the dry ingredients can be clumped together in your hand.
5. Pack the mixture into the muffin tin. Make sure to press the mixture tightly into the muffin tin.

6. Let the muffin tin sit for 10 minutes. During this time, lay a sheet of wax paper on top of a cookie sheet.
7. Turn the muffin tin over and carefully tap the bottom of the tin to encourage the bath bombs to carefully fall out and onto the wax paper.
8. Allow the bath bombs to dry overnight. When dry, carefully package them in small wedding favor boxes topped with a ribbon, the bride and groom's name and wedding date.

Itty Bitty Bath Bombs

Most bath bombs are really cute, but these itty bitty bath bombs take adorable to a whole new level. Give your friends and family a wonderful set of pebble-sized bath bombs.

Ingredients:

- 1 cup baking soda
- ½ cup citric acid
- ½ cup cornstarch
- 1 tablespoon baby oil
- ½ teaspoon witch hazel

- 1 teaspoon essential oil
- Food colouring
- Silicone ice cube mold

Directions:

1. Whisk the dry ingredients together in a bowl.
2. Whisk the baby oil, witch hazel and essential oil together in a different bowl.
3. Add one drop of food coloring at a time to the liquid ingredients. Stir after each drop. Continue until you have achieved the desired color.
4. Add the liquid ingredients to the dry ingredients a little at a time, quickly stirring after each bit is added.
5. Continue adding the liquid ingredients until the dry ingredients have the same consistency as damp sand and you can clump the mixture together in your hand.
6. Pack the mixture tightly into the silicone ice tray mold. Let the mixture sit in the molds for at least 4 hours but preferably overnight.

7. Carefully remove the bath bombs from the ice cube tray and store in an airtight container until ready to use.

Saturday Night Sizzle Bath Bombs

Add some extra sizzle to your bath before a night out on the town. This heavy mixture of scents gets you pumped up for a fantastic weekend.

Ingredients:

- 10 tablespoons baking soda
- 2 ½ tablespoons cornstarch
- 2 tablespoons tapioca starch
- 5 tablespoons citric acid
- 1 ½ tablespoons canola or sweet almond oil
- ½ teaspoon sodium lauryl sulfoacetate
- 2 to 3 drops of soap colorant
- 1 tablespoon essential or fragrance oil
- Witch hazel

Directions:

1. Sieve the dry ingredients together and into a large mixing bowl.

2. Mix the oil, sodium lauryl sulfoacetate, colorant and essential or fragrance oil together in another bowl.
3. Pour the liquid over the dry ingredients and mix together with your hands.
4. Spray the witch hazel lightly over the mixture and work it into the mixture. Continue lightly spraying the mixture with the witch hazel and mixing with your hands until it has the texture of damp sand.
5. Press the mixture into the mold and let sit for a few minutes.
6. Remove the bath bomb from the mixture and place on a cookie sheet covered with a fluffy towel. Allow the bath bombs to dry for 24 hours.

Manly Bath Bombs

People often consider bath bombs feminine because of the fragrances and colors, but this recipe gives the bath bombs a masculine combination of scents.

Ingredients:

- 2 tablespoons baking soda

- 1 tablespoon citric acid
- 1 tablespoon cornstarch
- 1 tablespoon Epsom salts
- ¼ teaspoon coconut oil
- ¾ teaspoon strong coffee
- Coffee grounds and walnuts, finely grounded
- Mini muffin tins

Directions:

1. Brew a strong cup of coffee. Let it cool to room temperature.
2. While the coffee is cooling, mix the baking soda, citric acid, cornstarch and Epsom salts in a bowl, using a whisk to achieve a fairly smooth consistency. Add finely ground coffee and walnuts to the mixture.
3. Mix ¾ teaspoon of the cooled coffee with the coconut oil in a small bowl.
4. Slowly pour the liquid mixture into the bowl of dry ingredients, whisking while you pour.
5. When the mixture starts feeling like damp sand, spoon the bath bomb mixture into

the mini muffin tins and press in tightly. Let them sit for about 4 hours.

6. Tap the bath bombs out of the mini muffin tins and leave to dry completely for 1 to 2 days.

Lots of Variations Bath Bombs

When it comes to bath bombs, variety is the name of the game. This recipe combines a wide range of scents and textures to give you a lot of variety packed into a single bath bomb.

Ingredients:

- ½ cup baking soda
- 2 tablespoons citric acid
- 1 tablespoon tapioca starch
- 2 tablespoons Shea butter, melted
- 5 drops each of peppermint, sage and lavender essential oil
- Spray bottle filled with witch hazel

Directions:

1. Mix the baking soda, citric acid and tapioca starch in a clean mixing bowl.

2. Combine the melted Shea butter and the essential oil in a separate bowl.
3. Drizzle the liquid mixture over the dry ingredients and use your hands to work the liquid into the dry mixture.
4. Use the spray bottle to spray the mixture lightly with the witch hazel. Mix with your hands after each spray, and continue until it can form clumps.
5. Press the damp sand-like mixture into the desired molds, letting it rest for a few minutes.
6. Turn the mold upside down and carefully tap the bath bombs out of the molds.
7. Set the bath bombs on a cookie sheet lined with wax paper and let harden for 24 to 48 hours.

Hard as Rock Bath Bombs

Although bath bombs are usually rock-solid after drying, this recipe takes it to a whole new level. These bath bombs store really well, and the beauty is that they dissolve and fizz in the tub just as easily as regular bath bombs.

Ingredients:

- 1 cup baking soda
- ½ cup citric acid
- ¼ cup Kaolin clay, also known as cosmetic clay
- ¼ cup sugar
- 1 large Vitamin E oil capsule or 2 small capsules
- 2 ½ tablespoons olive oil
- 1 tablespoon skin-safe fragrance oil or 20 drops essential oil
- 3 teaspoons water
- Colorant

Directions:

1. Mix the baking soda, citric acid and clay together in a mixing bowl.
2. Add one to two drops of the colorant to the dry mixture and knead with your hands.
3. Pour the water, olive oil and fragrance or essential oil into a spray bottle. Pierce the vitamin E capsule and dump the contents in the spray bottle.

4. Secure the lid on the spray bottle and shake vigorously for several seconds.
5. Spray the dry mixture with the liquid 1 to 2 times, kneading the mixture with your hands after every spray. Repeat this process until the mixture feels like damp sand.
6. Tightly pack the mixture into the desired molds. Wait a minute or two before tapping them out of the molds and onto a wax paper-lined cookie sheet.
7. Set the cookie sheet in a cool, dry location and let the bath bombs dry for 24 hours.

Fortune Cookie Bath Bombs

Fortune cookie bath bombs…why not? This recipe just shows how creative you can get. Have lots of fun making and using these lucky bath bombs.

Ingredients:

- 8 ounces baking soda
- 4 ounces citric acid
- 4 ounces cornstarch

- 4 ounces salts, such as Dead Sea salts, mineral salts or Epsom salts
- ¾ tablespoon water
- 2 tablespoons essential or fragrance oil
- 2 ½ tablespoons light oil
- 1 to 2 drops of food coloring
- Fortune cookie mold

Directions:

1. Mix together the dry ingredients ensuring that all lumps and clumps are removed.
2. Blend the liquid ingredients together in a small jar. If the jar has a lid, you can simply place the lid on top of the jar and shake for several seconds to thoroughly combine the wet ingredients.
3. Slowly add the wet ingredients to the dry ingredients while whisking. If the mixture begins to foam, you are adding the liquid too quickly. Slow down and remember to keep whisking.
4. Once you have added and mixed the wet and dry ingredients together, it should squish into a clump in your hand.

5. Press the bath bomb mixture into the fortune cookie mold. Let sit for several minutes before popping the bath bombs out of the mold and onto a wax paper-covered cookie sheet.
6. Allow the bath bombs to dry for 24 to 48 hours in a cool, dry location out of direct sunlight and away from direct heat.

BackToTop

Chapter 8: Conclusion

You can make making bath bombs a rewarding hobby for you. You can pack them for gifts or make it a business. It can also be a stress relieving activity. Nature walks can be a source of creativity. It can also be a fun activity with friends or family.

Above all, bath bombs are meant to be savoured and shared, and I hope with the help of this book, you've enjoyed doing both!

If you have truly found value in my publications please take a minute and rate my books, I'd be eternally grateful if you left a review on Amazon. As an independent author I rely on reviews for my livelihood and it gives me great pleasure to see my work is appreciated.

Lightning Source UK Ltd.
Milton Keynes UK
UKHW051842281218
334659UK00034B/493/P